MW01634912

# WHAT'S ABOVE?

BY KIM DENNIS

WITH KRISTA MACKINNON

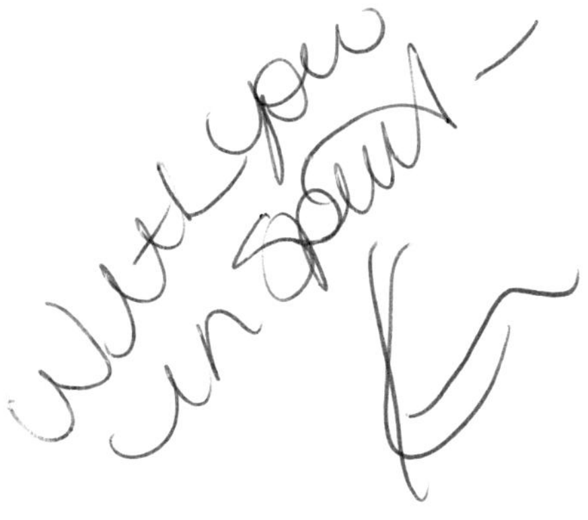

What's Above?



Co-Writer: Krista MacKinnon
Editor: Jason Anderson
Design: Krista MacKinnon

ISBN 0-9734193-0-X

Printed and bound in Canada.

For more information visit my website:
www.clairvoyantkim.com

Dedicated to

Ashley and Brenna

# Acknowledgements

Thank you to the many different souls that helped me create this book. Many people contributed, but without the advice of my publicist Andrea Christian, the support of the Singleton family and the editorial assistance of Jason Anderson, What's Above could never have been completed and presented in its current form.

My deepest gratitude goes to my friend Krista MacKinnon who, with her incredible talent and insight, helped me write this book. I thank her for all the long hours, hard work, dedication, inspiration and care. She truly believes in me and my work and for that I am eternally grateful. She saw the story in me long before I did and encouraged me to put it down on paper. She is truly the ultimate "ghost writer."

I am indebted to all those people who have come for readings over the years. Whether or not their stories are directly related in these pages, all of them are here. Special gratitude to those who generously allowed me to share their stories — without their time and their memories, this book would not be complete. Their stories will hopefully resonate with many people and provide greater insights and healing to others. They are the true heroes of this book.

Many thanks to my radio family — Christina Rowsell, Samantha Stevens, Tara Connors, Phil Kallsen, Patty MacNeil and Shannon Cooke — for believing in me and giving me the opportunity to share and help so many people on air. An extra special thanks to the late Pat O'Bryan, an incredible friend who gave me my first break in radio — may we all be so fortunate to meet someone as special and giving as him.

A special thanks to my family for their tremendous love and encouragement which helped me believe in what I do. Without your love, none of this would be possible.

# Contents

# 1

# The Journey

Before I even realized that I had fallen asleep, there He was. How could this be happening to me? Why was this happening to me?

No matter what questions or doubts flooded my mind at that moment, the truth was that Jesus was right there in front of me.

I had been watching *Coronation Street* when I dozed off into a light sleep. It was then that I had my vision of Jesus. So many thoughts whirled around in my head — I thought of everything and nothing all at once. My emotions became heightened. I felt both energized and peaceful at once. And no matter how hard I tried, I could not comprehend what was happening.

I could only see Him from the waist up. He looked exactly like he did in the pictures I had seen when I was young, with a short beard and long, wavy brown hair. The image that he presented of Himself may not have been what He looked like when He was alive but it was the one I would recognize.

I could hardly contain what I was feeling. I

was now in such disbelief that I could not trust my thoughts and emotions. I needed reassurance that this was actually happening so I asked Him who He was. He let me know He was Jesus. But when He spoke, He didn't use words. Instead, He filled me with his thoughts. His first message was more like a feeling of warmth and love. He patiently waited for me to take it all in. He then communicated to me everything was going to be all right. At that moment, I had never felt so alert, even though I was still asleep.

After He left, an angel appeared. From my prior experiences with the afterlife, I knew that angels were neither male nor female. Still, the presence of this angel felt feminine. All I could see was her glowing face and a few thick white bands of fabric that were continuously flowing all around her. Everything around us seemed peaceful and alive. I gained strength as she comforted me. She repeated that everything was going to be all right. I knew that it would be.

When I awoke from my vision, the episode of *Coronation Street* was just ending — the whole experience had lasted for almost half an hour yet seemed so quick. Even though it was such a fleeting moment, I never doubted what had happened. The experience was just too powerful.

I had hit a real low point in my life when this

happened. I was a single mother and I wasn't getting the help and support I needed. I was struggling financially and felt very alone. Before His visit, I had many feelings of anxiety and fear, feelings rooted in loneliness, hopelessness and despair.

I often wonder whether Jesus visited me because of the despair that I was feeling or if He had another reason. In either case, His visit was a real turning point in my life, one that helped me realize I was never alone. My vision confirmed my beliefs about God and gave me the strength to move my life in a new direction.

Most of the time, we go about our daily lives never thinking about what's around us. We hardly even notice other people when we walk or drive past them unless they do something annoying or extraordinary. Just think about how many times you have walked by a friend without recognizing him or her until one of you took a second look?

It is rare for us to give a second thought to anything outside our normal routines. Only in the event of a miracle or a tragedy are we inspired to really look around us. In our struggle to comprehend what has happened, we begin to ask questions about what's beyond this life. We may even ponder what's above.

I had already begun to ask myself these questions when I had my vision. "Is there a God?" I wondered. "Is there an afterlife? Are our loved ones that have passed on around us? If there is a God, then why does He not show himself to prove that He exists?" My visit from Jesus helped me build my beliefs on a firm foundation — God does exist and is around us all the time, trying to help.

But what if my experience had never happened? What if it was all a dream, only a product of my imagination? Would it still have altered the course of my life? Would my beliefs be any different? Would I still have become a medium?

I believe that I would have still discovered my gifts.

## Learning About God

There was nothing abnormal about my childhood. I had a nice typical upbringing in a nice suburban neighbourhood. We may not have had the kind of idealized family that existed only in 1950s sitcoms, but we all loved each other and tried to make a go of things.

Despite having supportive parents, my family could never have prepared me for becoming a medium. Even though I've since heard that my grandfather read teacups and that my great-grandmother had psychic powers, there certainly wasn't anyone I knew who was a practicing medium.

Many people would think that if I saw a

vision of Jesus then I must be religious or come from a religious family. But my family could hardly be described as religious. It wasn't that my family were adamantly atheistic — it was more that we did not practice any religion. The subject was rarely, if ever, discussed in my family.

Any ideas that I had about religion when I was young were influenced by my best friend Maureen. Her family lived across the street from my home. Maureen's family was Catholic and did not have much in common with my family so our parents barely knew each other. Maureen even went to a separate Catholic school so we met while playing in the neighbourhood after school. As soon as we did meet, we were inseparable.

Every Sunday, Maureen and her family went to church. Since we were not often apart on the weekends, I would wonder what she did there. Sometimes I asked her about it after she came home. Religion wasn't a regular topic of discussion for us but she would share what she learnt in Sunday school.

One thing she told me that really stuck with me was that if you ask for something from God, He would give it to you. Since I was only five years old at the time, I only tried it out on small requests. One evening, my mother told me I had a dentist appointment the next day. Like most children, I did not want to go. So as I was going to bed, I put out those thoughts of not wanting to go. When I woke up the next day, I discovered that the appointment had to be rescheduled. I was amazed that it worked.

In another incident, my mother and I spent what seemed like forever redecorating my bedroom with flower patterns and ruffles. I adored my grandmother and really wanted her to see it. Because my grandparents were elderly, we usually went to their home to visit so I never thought that she would ever be able to see it. When I drifted off to sleep that night, I thought about how wonderful it would be if she could see my room. To my surprise, my mother told me the next morning that my grandparents were coming for dinner. That night, I took great delight in showing Grandma everything we had done.

Soon enough, making these wishes became like a secret game. I would share all kinds of thoughts with God before I went to sleep and the next morning, things had a way of working out the way I wanted them to. I remember feeling so grateful to Maureen for sharing information about God. Looking back on this time, I now realize God put Maureen in my life so that I could get closer to Him.

## Discovering My Gifts

I first realized that there was something more to life than what we can see when I was eight years old. I began to have strange dreams in which I would hang between being awake and asleep. In these dreams, it seemed that there were things or people around me. When I told my mother about these dreams, she didn't seem concerned so I never gave them a second thought. After coming to me every so often over the next year, the dreams finally stopped one day.

When I was 13, stranger things began to happen. Feeling very tired from track-and-field practice, I came home from school one afternoon and went straight to bed. Before I realized what was happening, I felt my soul slip out of my body and just glide away. Rather than strange or extraordinary, it felt so natural for my soul to leave my body. I felt free and alive.

When I was released from the constraints of my body, my curiosity took over. I explored everything in my room, which felt like a whole new world. Everything seemed so quiet and peaceful — the feeling was way beyond what I could comprehend. The silence around me somehow enhanced all my other senses so what had been my ordinary bedroom ten minutes before took on a new and unreal quality.

As I started to move around the room, I became intrigued with my movements. It took me no time to get used to moving in all directions. It soon felt completely natural that I should be able to zoom up and down and every which way. At track-and-field practice that day, I would never have imagined that I could move at such speeds with grace and precision.

Throughout this time of discovery, I was conscious of what was around me. I saw my body below. I felt a twinge of fear that I might not be able to get back inside my body. This fear grew the longer I was away from it. I began to panic but there seemed to be nothing I could do to get back. Diving into my body didn't work. Neither did lying back down. I even tried to shake myself wake. I soon gave up trying but the fear never completely left me.

As I continued to move around my room, I was drawn toward a corner of the room. Whenever I paused, I would naturally start tumbling towards it. Something there wanted to take me further away. I had the feeling that it might open up and become as large as the universe itself. I was afraid to leave the confines of my room and lose sight of my body on the bed so every time I got near the corner, I would resist and pull back.

Suddenly, my mother opened the door to tell

me dinner was ready. I was immediately thrust back inside my body. It took a little while to adjust to being there again, but I soon shook off any dazed or drowsy feelings. When I tried to get out of bed, I became aware of the constraints placed on me by my body. It felt very cumbersome after the freedom I enjoyed only a few moments before.

I looked at my bedside clock and realized that the experience must have lasted two hours. In hindsight, I should have enjoyed the experience more but my fear of not being able to get back inside my body had been too great to thoroughly embrace it.

That first out-of-body experience provoked many questions for me. Why was I able to move around the room while my body stayed asleep on the bed below? What was in the corner and why did it feel like it was going to take me further away? I would relive the event again and again in my head, wondering how all this was possible. I also wondered whether it would happen again.

I did not have to wait long to find out. After falling into another light sleep a few days later, my soul again slipped out of my body, leaving me free to explore my room. Within a week of my first experience, I had three more. As I became more comfortable with the process, my fears subsided. When I realized I could get back inside my body whenever I wanted or needed to, it was no longer an issue. Soon I felt comfortable enough to even venture outside my room.

At first, I did not progress much further than my own house. But I soon progressed to travelling around my neighbourhood. As I explored, I would see things in real time. I could watch my Mom cook dinner or the other kids as they played in the neighbourhood. When I talk about it now, the whole experience takes on a fantastic quality but everything felt very real. Because my senses were so heightened, I saw my home and my neighbourhood in a way that was more fully alive than I did when I was awake. Even the smallest things had more depth and shape — a pebble in the road became something extraordinary to behold.

My first out-of-body experience seemed to unlock a door. Soon, it was happening on a daily basis. Whenever I fell into a light sleep or took a nap in the middle of the day, I was sure to travel outside my body. These experiences lasted for almost a decade and were strongest between the ages of 19 and 23.

My first out-of-body experience was hugely important to me — until then, I didn't even know if there was a God. At first my experiences would consist of venturing out and exploring everything in a haphazard way. Gradually I became aware of a guide who would on some occasions show me and teach me things. I knew that I had known this soul for a very long time but once I woke up, I was no longer able to remember who it was. It was as if my mind went blank whenever I wanted to think of him. Since I was only 13, my thoughts were confused.

Though I did not realize it at first, he was there with me all the time, showing me what I needed to learn. I would see him most clearly when I was being taken to a higher plane. He had pale green eyes and was very, very tall. He would show me more and more.

**2**

# Gaining Knowledge

As soon as I left my body, I was in heaven. But within heaven there are different levels. Being around my family in our house or in the neighbourhood is only one part. The heaven that most people think of as heaven is on a higher plane. About a year after my first out-of-body experience, I started to travel there.

During that first time, I worried that I had died. But my guide helped me overcome my fears and explore. Even after travelling there with my guide, I am not sure what or where it is but it felt like the place that people go when they pass over. I saw images of people I knew who had passed on — my father's parents, my aunt Doris. I also saw many children who I did not recognize but told me they were my mother's brothers and sisters. When I did a family tree many years later, I discovered that my grandmother had 19 pregnancies but only gave birth to nine children.

The first few times that I travelled to heaven, I was shown beautiful gardens. They looked similar to some of the fabulous gardens here on Earth except that everything was so much more alive — the sky, the animals, the plants, even the colours exuded a vibrancy that I had never seen before and have never seen since. I saw everything in a way that isn't possible for our eyes on earth. The depth and lustre of the colours seemed to have an energy and life force all to themselves. Until you see red and green in heaven, you cannot even begin to understand what they are.

Whenever I entered heaven, I was overwhelmed by unconditional love, joy, happiness, laughter, serenity, peace and many more wonderful feelings. Somehow all the negativity that we experience in this world just does not exist there. These strong new feelings were neither thrust upon me, nor exactly "felt." It was more like they were all around me as something I both knew and felt.

After a couple of visits, I began to understand why I was there. Part of it was to share in the love, joy and beauty that existed there. Another reason was to show me that it was nothing to be feared. In time I realized that by experiencing heaven, I could help those who were left behind to know their loves ones have truly gone to a better place.

You should not feel bad for those that pass over because they are the lucky ones. Once a loved one passes over, any illness or deformity instantly disappears. The truth is that we never truly die: our bodies are left behind as our souls continue on.

I also learnt that there is no judgement in heaven. God does not judge you — instead, you judge yourself. The guide showed me that after we finish our lives, we follow a bright light to the other side and go into what appears to be a classroom. There, we watch our lives on TV screens. Everything we did throughout our lives has been captured. When we watch it, not only do we see our lives but we feel every moment as well.

One startling discovery for me was that besides seeing and feeling our lives again, we also feel everything that we made others feel. That is why it is so important to help others and to treat them like you would want to be treated. Otherwise, what you do will catch up with you in heaven and you will have to relive it from the perspectives of those you hurt.

I do not know how many times I visited heaven but I saw enough to understand how wonderful it will feel when I go back home to stay.

## Denial

When I shared these experiences with close family members and friends, most could not relate to what I was saying. My mother and my aunt Donna did not know what to make of it. Others gave me questioning looks. Since I could not adequately explain how or why this was happening to me, I tried to put what was happening to me out of my mind.

When I was in my twenties, I went through what I call my "intuition" phase. I developed the ability to automatically know things that there was no way that I could have known.

When this first began to happen, I attributed my insights to being sensitive to what other people were thinking. Up until around the time I had my first daughter when I was 23, this seemed to be a reasonable explanation. However, over the following 12 years, the sixth sense grew stronger and stronger and my insights became greater and greater. I eventually had to reassess what was happening to me.

There was a game I played in the time I worked at a bank. Being a teller, I would spend most of my day waiting on customers. From where I was standing, I could not see the parking lot, but a name or face would sometimes pop into my head. I would then either write down the name on a piece of paper or tell my co-workers. Usually within a few minutes, I would see that person walk through the door.

At first, this just seemed to be an innocent guessing game. Whenever I was right, I attributed it to coincidence — it seemed so natural that I would know this. When it started to occur more regularly and my guesses consistently proved correct, my co-workers thought that it was a magic trick. They would constantly ask me how I did it. I realized I had no idea myself. This was unsettling but I didn't want to face the possibility that my talent might be something more.

I also began to have more insights into events or people. Once, when I was talking to a friend on the telephone, I interrupted our conversation to ask if she had cut her finger. After a long pause, she replied that she had cut her finger earlier that morning. "How did you know?" she asked.

Soon, this sort of thing was happening constantly. I would know who was calling me or who was at the door. I would know what people were thinking or what had happened to them. Sometimes I would even know what was going to happen before it happened. After I told people the thoughts that kept popping into my head, they questioned me about how I could know these things. I could not blame them for asking because I was also baffled.

As time went on, people's questions bothered me more and more. I was nagged by questions: why was this happening to me? How did it work? I felt very uneasy and alone. I finally reached a point where I tried to forget about all of this, but the more I ignored it, the stronger my insights became.

Coincidences were happening all the time. One Sunday morning I got my young daughter into the car and dashed to the grocery store. Just as I drove into the parking lot, I had a passing thought about a couple I had known years ago in Ontario. I quickly forgot about them as I found a parking spot and helped my daughter out of the car. Sure enough, I saw the couple I was thinking about as soon as we entered the store. I was so stunned that I almost dropped my daughter. I had experienced many coincidences before but this was a moment that convinced me I really had to listen to what was going on around me.

After I realized that this ability was not going away, I finally accepted that I had something special that made me different from other people. Since I still didn't know what it was or what I should do with it, I did the only thing that I could do: I surrendered to God. I looked up to the sky and said, "There is something going on here. I do not know what this is. I do not know what to do with this. Show me the way."

From that point on, I was just shown what to do on each and every day. I just accepted. I was reluctant to say I was psychic but I did become more accepting of the possibility.

I soon had another life-changing moment. Up until this time, I had never heard of people communicating with the other sides except for stories about séances and Ouija boards. Then one day I had the TV on while I was busy with housework. The Oprah Winfrey show came on and her guest was the medium Rosemary Altea. I was glued to the TV and swiftly put a tape in the VCR to record it. I had never before seen someone connecting with spirit and everything she said about her experiences with the other side resonated with me. It was such a relief to know that someone else had these experiences. As soon as the show was over, I went out and bought Rosemary's latest book. I couldn't put it down.

It was also around this time that I saw Jesus. His visit did more for me than I will ever realize. His visit itself let me know that He existed and that I was never alone. I needed a sign that I was right to trust in God and His visit confirmed it. He gave me the strength to continue.

Bit by bit I was pointed in the right direction. I genuinely felt that I could help others by becoming a medium and everything began to fall into place to make that happen. I seemed to draw in the right books, the right information and the right people to start to use my talents.

**Developing My Gift**

One day, a flyer from a Spiritualist church was delivered to my door. Before receiving this, I hadn't known that Spiritualist churches existed — there was even one right in my neighbourhood. I began attending church every Sunday. I was unsure about what to expect but I found that they helped me understand what was happening. I felt very relieved that I wasn't weird and that I wasn't alone in my feelings. They helped me focus and develop my innate talents.

I also attended a meditation class for an hour one night a week for a year. In each class, five to six people would sit in a circle and share energies. First, a prayer would be said. Then we would spend 20 minutes trying to clear our heads and listening for messages for ourselves and for others in the group. At the end of each session, we would go around the room to see if we had any messages for each other.

The class helped me focus and allowed me to practice setting aside my thoughts so that I could listen to the spirits around me. This may sound simple but you'd be surprised about how difficult it is to achieve. I had great difficulty separating my thoughts from what was being said. I needed to quiet myself on the inside and empty my thoughts.

Through the church, I learnt that anyone can

communicate with spirits, although some people find it more difficult than others. Most people had the same problem as I did with quieting their thoughts. Basically, to listen, we need to stop thinking. When people start to hear spirits, most messages are about themselves. Once you can listen for yourself, you can then listen for others. That was what I wanted to achieve.

After a year of practising with the group, I could focus without their help. Clearing your mind is such a huge part of communicating with spirits so I would recommend to anyone wanting to try it to keep practising and not to get frustrated when it does not happen right away. The key is to stop looking outside for answers — go within. As Oprah Winfrey says, "The noise of the world will drown out the voice of God; you have to be quiet within yourself to listen."

The journey of discovering and exploring my gifts was one I had to take by myself. My close friends may have known about my gift, but for the most part, they did not know what to think. They weren't frightened by it and some even told me I should do something with it, but only as a passing statement. Still, they weren't surprised when I became a medium.

Unfortunately, I also did not get much help from my family through this process. Even though my mother was interested, she did not understand what was happening. Considering that I did not understand it either, there was not much she could have done.

I realized the truth in something else Oprah Winfrey has said: "On the road to success you'll lose some friends along the way." As I became more successful, some of my closest friends — people I had known for over 20 years — turned their backs on me.

After my first radio program aired, I was so thrilled to share it with my friends that I brought a recording of my show to one of our regular get-togethers. When I told them about being on the radio and started to play the tape, I felt so hurt when they weren't excited — one friend even walked out of the room barely after I had started to play it. I had wanted them to be happy for me and for what I had been able to accomplish. Sadly, it just did not turn out that way.

Some friends may have left my life, but new ones were drawn in. As I changed and grew, I found myself in new situations that allowed me to meet new people who have been extremely supportive and helpful. I now have an overwhelming number of people that I can call true friends. I feel truly blessed.

## Overcoming Fallacies

After becoming a medium, I really struggled with the concept of "fortune telling" being attached to what I do: how can I know the future? And if that future is known, how can it be changed? When people came for readings, they often wanted to know what would happen to them over the course of their entire lifetime. I firmly believe that we change our lives through our choices, but if that is true, I should not be able to predict what will happen to people. At times, I felt like a hypocrite, saying to people that they can change their lives in one breath and then in the next, telling them that all this will happen.

I have tried to resolve this dilemma by reading books, meditating and speaking to the other side, but I still do not completely understand it. However, I do know there is no such thing as fortune telling. Certain things may happen for certain reasons but overall, we create our own destinies. Every step we take steers us toward a different outcome so we need to choose our path carefully. Our perspective here is so limited but people on the other side can see the bigger picture. We see our lives like a movie that is only partly finished — spirits and God can see the whole thing. They can even see different outcomes depending on the choices we make. Having this knowledge allows them to "predict" what will happen on our current path.

Another thing that bothered me along the way was the power of suggestion. It is so huge. At times, I do not like to say what will happen to people because each person has the power to make that suggestion a reality. Personally, I find it a very fine line between what is predetermined and what is by our own making. The only way that I can continue to do readings for people is to know that it is through God that I get these messages. He is the one that gives me the information and I only give people the information that I get. Without that knowledge, I would not be willing to take on the responsibility that comes with doing readings.

As my abilities have become stronger, I find it much easier to talk with souls whenever and wherever I am. Many people ask me if I find this a huge burden. My only response is that it comes so naturally to me that I would find it strange if I could not communicate with the other side. Besides, I do not speak with spirit all the time — I can pull it in and push it out.

I remember a recent incident when I was at a nightclub with a group of friends. As we were sitting at the table, the spirit of a father came to me. I quickly glanced around the table. All of my friends' fathers were still alive so I put it out of my mind and continued to enjoy one of my rare evenings out. Later that night, one friend came back with someone I had met at a radio station party. I remembered that her father had passed away. The spirit told me he died of prostate cancer. Out of the blue, I asked this woman if this was how her father died. She confirmed that this was the case. Since we were having such a nice time, I left it at that, but the incident just confirmed to my friends that souls are constantly around me.

Some of my friends feel sorry for me because I cannot escape from souls vying for attention. Since they know the presence of spirits sometimes give me an itchy nose, my friends believe there is a spirit around whenever I scratch it. I constantly have to tell them that sometimes an itchy nose is just an itchy nose.

# 3

## Answers To Life's Questions

Who am I? Why am I here? Where is my place in the world or even the universe? These are just a few of the questions we all ask ourselves. While I do not have all the answers, what I have learnt through my out-of-body experiences and communicating with souls will hopefully provide some guidance and reassurance.

Some of the most difficult questions concern God. Does He exist? Did He create us? Where is He? I once heard God described not as the thought to move your arm or the arm's movement but the spark in your brain that connects the two. He is the reflex to breathe, the beat of your heart. He is simply what makes us alive.

Some people may use a different name than "God." That's what I prefer because people can relate to it and understand He is the source of life. Whatever you choose to call it, it is what it is: a universal energy.

I believe that everyone and everything is connected through God. God flows through everything — from plants and animals to each one of us. Even

some things that we may not consider living —
such as a table and chairs — are connected to him.
There is absolutely nothing in which God does not
exist. And when we learn how His energy works, we
can use it to make wonderful things happen in our
lives.

I believe that each of us consist of two main
parts. One is our physical bodies, which are the
shells or containers for us here on Earth. The other
is our souls, which live forever. God is present in
both parts.

Our understanding of the universe resides in
our souls. While we are on Earth, we can only tap
into a small portion of that knowledge. All of us
have had many lives. Our souls are timeless, but
just like schoolchildren in different grades, we are
each at different stages and learn at our own paces.

Our souls play a major role in predetermining
aspects of our life. Our souls not only choose when
we come into this world and when we leave but
also the basis of what type of lives we're going to
lead. Depending on what we need to experience,
our souls choose our parents, and thus some of the
physical and personality characteristics we will
inherit. For instance, if you want to be an Olympic
athlete, you choose parents who will pass on the
athletic attributes you need. If you want to be a
comedian, you will choose parents who will pass on

aspects of that family's personality to enable you to achieve that life.

The reason why our souls come down here at all is to learn. Our souls are works-in-progress. I like to think of the world as a big university campus where we all take different classes. Sometimes, a single class will take a lifetime to complete. Or we might take many different classes over a single lifetime. We may even choose to repeat some classes to try different outcomes. Learning never ends, so as soon as we have finished one lesson, there is another one waiting for us.

No matter what the lesson may be, it is important to know that we are all here for a purpose. We all have certain things that we want to learn and experience. While some lessons may appear similar, the experiences and outcomes are as individual as we are. As we move through our lives, we draw in people who help facilitate those goals.

Even though our lives may seem somewhat predetermined, we still have choices. Once we come down here, we have a rough idea about what we want to learn. It is through our choices that we learn those life lessons. The path we take can be smooth or rough, depending on how we choose. We create our own destinies.

God gave us free will. If we don't like the directions of our lives, we need to do something to change them. God will not magically make it happen for us.

Fortunately, God will help us if we want to change our paths. He will give you opportunities to change, but if you choose not to act, nothing will happen.

At times, the world may not make sense to us. We must remember that we don't have all the information we need. Depending on what a soul has chosen to learn, she or he will have different experiences. Some experiences will be wonderful and happy while others will seem terrible and unfair. Until our lives here ends, we won't truly understand the purpose and meaning behind both joyful and painful experiences.

When they do pass over, our souls leave our bodies behind. We still retain every experience we had while living and we still care about the families and friends who we knew. Sometimes it may seem wrong for people to die when they do but please remember that our souls choose when they want to come into this world and when to leave. No one goes before her or his time.

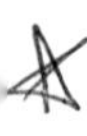

Furthermore, we all go to heaven. No matter what your particular faith or the type of a person you were on Earth, we all travel towards the light and enter the gates of heaven. And once you are there, nobody judges you except yourself. When I visited heaven, I watched souls that had just passed away go into a room with what seemed to be mini-TVs. Each soul found a spot and then reviewed its life. Not only did they relive each moment, but they also felt how they made others feel. Our lives are not about what we achieve. Instead, they are about giving. These are the moments that define our lives.

Once your soul is in heaven, all of the boundaries and limitations of this world are removed. Your current way of thinking about time and space does not exist. Heaven has no beginning and no end — it defies all earthly measurements. When I am communicating with souls, it is difficult to get a timeline from them — up there, they lose all sense of it.

Once these constraints are lifted, our souls can travel and be numerous places instantly. I do not know if they can be in more than one place at a time but I do know that they can travel at the speed of thought. When I am doing a telephone reading, the other person can put a thought out there and within moments I can get the answer. I like to think of it as a sort of paging system. If you think about them or if you need their help, then put that thought out there and they will be there.

A few unfortunate souls either don't know that they've passed over or know where to go. Generally all they really need is a reminder. If you tell them that family and friends who have already passed are waiting for them on the other side, then you won't see them again.

I encountered a soul like this shortly after I started to perform readings. I was living in a big, old house with my two children. My oldest child told me several times that she could hear me opening the front door and walking down the hall when she was in the basement. She mentioned this more than once so I knew it must have been bothering her.

Not long afterwards, my oldest child was away at school and I was with my youngest child in her room when we heard the front door open. The closet door opened and footsteps could be heard moving along the short hall. The footsteps continued past the room that we were in but no one appeared in the open doorway. Instead they continued into a spare room. My youngest thought it was her older sibling but I knew that the footsteps were not hers. Not even a shadow had passed the open doorway. As soon as I heard the spirit walking down the hall, I realized what it was and my maternal instincts took over.

Wanting to protect my daughter, I went into the spare room. Rather than feel afraid of what was going on, I was upset that my children were being frightened. I confronted the spirit. "I don't know who you are," I said, "and I don't think that you mean any harm but you're scaring my kids. I think you're lost but you need to know that your loved ones are waiting for you. And if you ever want to visit me, then please come and talk to me but please don't scare my children."

We never heard from that soul again.

## Messages From The Other Side

Even though souls go to heaven, they don't forget about their friends and family still on Earth. They still care about us and want to help us. They will even try to communicate with us in subtle ways. They could be in the form of a passing thought or a familiar smell, like a whiff of apple pie. Generally, it will appear and disappear just as swiftly. This is their way of letting you know that they are around you.

Whenever you want your loved ones to come around you, just ask either out loud or by putting that thought out. They are more than happy to come. When they visit you, they can surround you with healing energies. Even those of us on Earth can send out healing energies, but you may prefer the warmth of someone you've lost.

Even though souls lose the restrictions that we have on Earth, they still only have limited powers to help us. If you can clear your mind or know how to meditate, you can listen for their advice or words of comfort. But for real change, insights or guidance, it is best to ask for God's help.

It is a nice idea that our grandmothers or beloved uncles could be our guardian angels but angels are different than us. They have never had lives on Earth. We have lives on Earth so that we can learn what they already know. When God allowed us to come down here, He didn't just leave us and hope for the best. He allowed angels and other souls to help us.

He also allows us to tap into a small portion of the knowledge we have as souls by giving us our inner voices. I like to think of the inner voice as not only the voice of our souls but also the voice of God. Whenever you listen to your inner voice, you are listening to God's guidance. That voice can help you throughout your life, helping with decisions both big and small. It could be anything from whether you should turn left or right at an intersection to whether you should marry someone. Our inner voices will always help us make the right decisions. You do not need to guess your way through life. By listening to your inner voice and praying to God, He will help you.

It may be difficult to trust your inner voice but it is always right. In life, we need to think less and feel more. I constantly hear people talking about how when they were listening to someone, a voice from inside them told them the opposite of what they were hearing was true. We need to have faith that our inner voice can always be trusted to help us do the right thing.

One way to listen better to your inner voice is to learn to mediate.  We get so involved with our lives, we become anxious and can't listen to any-thing. Meditation is about quiet listening, a time when we can let go of all the mind's chatter and lis-ten to our souls and to God.

Choosing a time and place for meditation is very important. I find that meditating in the early morning is best. At that time, I am the only one awake in my household and it is still quiet outside. I make a cup of tea and I sit on the couch in the dark. I let go of my thoughts and become quiet with myself. From my inner voice, I gain insights into everything from the smallest of details to the biggest things. Let your inner voice guide you through these moments. It already knows all your concerns so be patient and allow your inner voice to tell you what is important and what is not.

Even if you ignore your inner voice, your soul will try to communicate to us through thoughts that you have during the day. Any recurring thought is a message from your soul. Sometimes it is obvious to everyone except ourselves. One time, a young girl came with her mother for a reading. "What should I do as a career?" she asked me. I immediately had a vision of a sewing machine so I asked her about it. She explained that she had been sewing since she was 7. She could sew almost anything but it was just a hobby. It had never occurred to her that she should choose a career based on her lifelong passion. She was making it difficult on herself by not listening. Eventually she did listen to her inner voice and started her own company that makes wedding dresses. She has since told me that it does not feel like work. In fact, she can't believe that people are paying her to have so much fun. When you find something that you enjoy, you're usually on the right path.

Amazing growth can be achieved when our souls and our personalities are in synch. By listening to your inner voice, you can hear where your soul wants to direct you. If your personality starts to travel in that same direction, then you are unstoppable. You can accomplish amazing things and live the best possible life. You can achieve a fulfilling and powerful life.

Many people who contact me for readings are not happy in their lives. Some who appear to have it all still feel that something is missing. We may believe that if we have success and money then we'll be happy. Generally, the missing element is generosity with others. Not surprisingly, I rarely hear schoolteachers or people in the service industry express these feelings. But many people feel their work lacks meaning.

Not everyone is meant to be a teacher, but somewhere in these people's chosen career paths, they may have doubted themselves and chosen what they thought they should do rather than what they wanted to do. Even though they chose a different path, people can still follow their inner voice. People always have a perception that life decisions are all or nothing — instead, they are about taking small steps. Even if you do not know exactly what you want, just take one step in a new direction. Keep taking small steps in that direction until you hit a brick wall, then move in a different direction. When everything falls into place, you know you've made the right decision. It is not going to be perfect along the way, but if that is the direction you're meant to go in, it will work out.

Sometimes even people who have found meaning in their chosen paths feel that something is missing. Suddenly, everything seems terribly wrong. Whenever this happens we need to look at what we give to those around us.

We receive what we put into life. This cycle is called karma. Think of karma as a circle. Anything that we do unto others will be done unto us.

Everything that we make other people feel will come right back to us either from that same person or even from someone else.  No deed, good or bad, goes unnoticed — everything has an effect. For instance, every time that we help someone, we will get something positive back. However if we make someone feel bad, something bad will come back at us. In short, nobody gets away with anything. Everything comes full circle.

The easiest way to gain what we need is to give it away. If we want more love, then give love away. If we want more money, then give money away. Every moment of every day is a chance to change our karma. We can change our karma when we wake up. Or we could start our lives anew with each breath.

Even though we can change our karma instantly, our karma from the past will still have to be played out — we cannot erase everything that we have done. But as soon as we start to give or help people, positive energy will be drawn into the cycle. By continuing to go in that new direction, we will create a new karma cycle. New energy will come back at us, enriching our lives.

# 4

## Insights Into A Reading

Not everyone understands how mediums are able to give insights into the lives of others. It seems extraordinary that we can communicate with the other side. When I do a reading, what happens is that I channel through to the souls connected to each person who has passed away. But this explanation leaves people with many questions: How and why souls are around us? How does a medium like myself channel or communicate with them?

When souls go to heaven, they are not in a confined place. Rather they are free to continue to help, guide and care for us from the other side. Souls are still connected to us through the experiences we shared and through God. Even though they may not be here living their lives with us any more, we have not lost them.

Whenever someone who has lost a friend or family member comes to me for a reading, I find that he or she is searching for a way to know that this loved one lives on. By sharing a reading, I give people proof.

One of the easiest ways for me to explain how

I communicate to souls is to describe what happens before, during and after a reading. I hope this chapter alleviates fears and answers questions about what I do.

Prior to a reading, I will usually pick up on some of the souls around the person coming even before he or she arrives. This may happen when I do something as simple as reading the person's name in my day-timer.

About 10 to 20 minutes before the person arrives, I take some time to say a few prayers. I say a prayer to thank God for everything that He has done for me and as to thank Him for the gift He has given me. I also say one for the person who is coming for the reading. I ask God to give me the guidance to help him or her and give the messages that he or she needs.

I find that many people are anxious when they arrive. They may be feeling uneasy about confronting the unknown or nervous about the messages they may receive. People tend to have a preconception of what I should look like. Sometimes they are surprised that I am not in my sixties — one lady who had arrived for a reading even asked me if my mother was home. Others say they expected me to be fat, or ugly and withered like a witch in a movie. Some people imagine that I look like a gypsy or an old fortune-teller from a country fair.

But when they see a small blond woman opening the door, most people are instantly put at ease.

As soon as someone comes in, I give him or her some time to relax and settle in on the couch with a warm cup of tea. When someone makes an appointment, the person generally has some questions in mind so I encourage him or her to ask me about anything. Not everyone who has a reading is at a pivotal point in their lives, but the ones that do ask many questions about their lives and life in general. Others may have a great desire to know what has happened to loved ones who have passed away and to feel that they are not alone. These people come from all walks of life with varying levels of understanding.

If someone has been referred to me, he or she usually knows already that I speak to the souls around them. Still, some are taken aback when I explain this. Even though many people are comforted to hear from loved ones, some find it difficult. They find it especially frustrating that they are unable to reach out to loved ones like they did when they were alive.

To start a reading, I sit in my chair and relax. I let go of my thoughts and listen to what the souls are saying to me. Souls and spirits are around all of us all the time, but they come in closer during a reading so that I can hear them better. They do not take over my body or anything like that — it is more like I am simply listening to a conversation. If at any point I need to ask them anything, I put the question out there either by saying it out loud or by saying it in my head. The souls can also hear and react to what other people in the room are saying and thinking so if they ask me any questions, I will sometimes have a reply before they finish asking me.

People are often shocked when I first start a reading. If they came with a need to reach someone who has passed away, then usually those souls speak to me first and help answer specific questions. The only real exception to this is when someone has passed away recently. A soul that has just finished a life seems to need time to rejuvenate, especially when that person may have been suffering from a long illness before dying.

At the beginning of every reading, I feel a surge of energy around me this indicates there is more than one soul around. Souls are anxious to talk to us and they come around me for a specific person. For instance, they will know that someone will get through to me on the radio before that person may even have thought to call the show. It is only when I start talking to that specific person that I discover why that soul has been around me.

All the souls want to speak at once. After 30 to

40 minutes, they have said what they need to. Sometimes when the information is coming at me very quickly, I need to interrupt people so that I can pass on all of the details.

To make sure that I am correctly understanding what is being said to me by a spirit, I ask the people in the room for yes-or-no answers after I repeat what I am being told. Whenever I get a no, I ask the soul for more information or for clarification. Usually the new information makes sense to the person or at least gives them enough to ask other relatives. They might be able to provide a better insight into that soul or the situation being discussed. After readings, many people will ask relatives about what they have been told about those on the other side — people in their twenties are not as aware of people who have passed. Though a younger person who comes for a reading may be worried about no one showing up, everyone has someone who has passed.

During a reading, information just starts to flow. It is as if I can hear a different frequency than the one on which people usually communicate. It is like an antenna that picks up a higher vibration or an animal that can hear sounds out of the range of our hearing.

When I am on the radio or doing a reading by telephone, the energy of the souls for each person will come around me. It may be hard for us to conceive how our souls are limitless but we need to remember that we're the ones that have boundaries. We are limited by time and space. When I am doing a reading, I do not need to have that person in front of me because I am reading the souls around him or her.

Since everything is connected to God, it is through Him that messages are then passed to me. The energy of the souls on the other side does most of the work. When I connect to them, it is just like hearing people talk. They feed me all the information that I need. Since I work with them all the time, they know when to give me a lot of information and when to give me little pieces.

About half the time I do readings, I can actually see the soul's energy. The energy looks like a grey-and-white cloud that travels like a wisp of smoke would, floating and flowing through the room. When this happens, I can follow their movements. Sometimes I can see faces, but it is difficult to distinguish what I see from what they are telling me. When I describe how someone looks, it is usually how the person would have looked to the person receiving the reading or to other family members who knew them. They come in that form so that they can be recognized but they do not look like that any more.

When all the souls that arrived for that person have had a chance to say their messages, they start to move away from me. I can tell when a reading has come to an end when they have all moved away and their conversations have died down. They do not exactly leave — they just fade out until they have pulled back completely. It is also at this point that most people will say, "Well, you have answered all my questions."

## Trial And Error

I performed my first reading for someone from the Spiritualist church. This woman was at a pivotal point in her career and wanted to find out more about it. Throughout the reading, I was very nervous and unsure about what I was supposed to do. I ended up sitting on the couch and saying whatever thoughts came to me. Fortunately I was able to pick up quite a few things about her going into business for herself.

When the reading was over, she was quite surprised at how well I did. She was the perfect person for my first reading because she had gone to the Spiritualist church and had an understanding of what I was doing.

After that reading, my business started to grow. People found out about me mainly through word-of-mouth from others who had come to see me. I also noticed that the more readings I performed, the stronger my gift became.

In the following chapters, you will read about people I have helped through my readings. Names have been changed and some stories have been slightly altered to protect people's privacy. I hope you are inspired by them and they help you become more attuned to the other side.

5

# Revelations

I first met Victoria when she came for a reading two years ago. Her reading taught me to trust what I was getting and to see what kind of impact my insights could have in people's lives.

Before I even met Victoria, I met her mother. Her mother was as anxious as a child waiting for Christmas morning. She could not wait to talk to me, and especially to Victoria. Though her daughter's appointment was not until late in the evening, she showed up 12 hours earlier. During that time, her mother kept asking to talk to me. I had to explain that I was busy tidying the house and doing laundry and would speak to her later.

When Victoria arrived for a reading, her mother was ready to burst. She could hardly wait for Victoria to come in and sit down.

"Was it your mother that you wanted to talk to?" I asked, knowing that her mother was anxiously awaiting my attention.

Victoria was a bit taken back by my question. She smiled and replied in a soft voice, "She passed away nine years ago."

Her mother did not want to waste any more time and everything that had been building up all day began to gush out. She described where Victoria worked down to the tiniest details, such as the material used for the cabinetry. She even described what Victoria saw from behind the counter.

Her mother then showed me a baby boy who was connected to Victoria's husband. Victoria looked at me with a blank expression, unable to place what I was saying.

"The name he is giving me is Henry," I told her.

Victoria still did not know who it was. Nevertheless, he kept coming up throughout the reading — he even showed me that he hadn't been alive when he was born. Victoria still shook her head. Finally, I asked her to ask her mother-in-law after the reading was over.

Another soul that showed up around her mother was her aunt Mary. Victoria was a bit confused because her aunt was still alive. I explained that she had cancer. Victoria pondered this for a while and recalled that her aunt did have breast cancer but the information still didn't click with her. I left it with her and moved on.

When we were on a completely different topic in the middle of the reading, her mother spoke up again. She told me that her name was Louise. Victoria suddenly had a huge adrenaline rush — she couldn't stop shaking. Victoria had taken special care not to tell me her mother's name so when I said it, she couldn't believe it. She later confessed that she had been stunned by the accuracy of the details during the reading and was afraid that she wouldn't be able to absorb everything that I had said. By the time she left, she felt overwhelmed.

However, this was only the beginning of the story. When she started to investigate the things that I said that had confused her, Victoria's experience moved to a higher level. When she went home that evening, she asked her husband about Henry, but he had no idea who that could be. The following morning, he asked his mother. When she heard the name, she nearly dropped her coffee.

Victoria's husband had an older brother who was ten years older. But there had also been a stillborn child, who arrived a year after the older brother's birth. In those days, a stillborn child had to have a proper name if the parents wanted a Protestant burial. His mother had chosen Henry. She had been told that she would never have children again after his birth but she did have an unexpected surprise nine years later.

After discovering that revelation, Victoria called her father to tell him about her experience.

She asked him about her aunt Mary. She could not understand how Mary had shown up because, as her father confirmed, she was still alive. However, her father was able to piece it together. Her mother had a friend of the same name who Victoria had called "Aunt Mary." This Mary had only passed away about a month before the reading. Both Mary and her husband had been close friends with Victoria's parents and lived close by. Her father had even worked with Mary's husband in the radio business for a number of years. Given that she was a close friend of her mother, that explained why Mary had shown up beside her mother.

## New Opportunities

Another important set of revelations came out of that first reading concerned Victoria's husband. He was out of work and she was wondering if there were any opportunities for him on the horizon. Her mother helped me describe some jobs she saw him doing. There were images of him around trees and then metal machinery — might he become a tree specialist or a machinist? I also understood something about him getting temporary work in the north. I felt that it wasn't a northern country or city, but rather in the northern part of Calgary. The last detail was that he would soon get a job that would take him overseas, a change that would have a major impact on their finances.

Two days later a friend called Victoria's husband to ask him to help on his landscaping projects — all of those projects were on the north side of Calgary. Shortly thereafter, another friend told Victoria's husband about an eight-month job in Russia. This job completely pulled them out of financial debt.

Just before the end of our reading, we had one more visitor. The young man wasn't coming into focus so I felt that she didn't know him very well. He explained that he was doing some type of mountain sport when he had a fatal accident. Victoria realized that this was Lee, a young man she had worked with at a ski shop ten years earlier. Her last contact with him was two months before he died. He had been skiing at Whistler when he tried to jump over a road but did not have enough momentum.

He came through to say hello and to ask Victoria to let his mother know that he is all right. When Victoria told his mother, she said that she wasn't brave enough to visit me but she did get sensations of Lee being around her.

## A New Perspective

Victoria calls her reading "the most amazing experience of my life." It also helped her start to piece together her beliefs about life and death.  When she was young, her mother attended a Swedenborgian church every Sunday with the family. When they moved to Calgary when Victoria was 11, their new city didn't have a church like it and the family stopped practicing.

"I was too young to really form any real understanding about God," Victoria says now. Her mother had tried to teach her but she wasn't able to tune in. What happened during our reading made sense to her because some of it was very much in accordance with her mother's beliefs.

Victoria had a very difficult time with her mother's illness and passing. She had quite a few regrets about the way that she handled things. Throughout her reading, Victoria realized that her mother forgives her for the way she acted before her death and that she loves her unconditionally.

After learning that she has not completely lost her loved ones, Victoria also found it much easier to deal with death. The anniversary of her mother's passing was no longer so difficult for her.

**6**

## Faith Prevails

Roy's mother had died a year before he and his wife Yvette came to see me. This was not the first time they tried to contact her. A few months before, another medium had come to their house but they were disappointed with the results. This left Roy further depressed over his inability to reach his mother. He badly needed to know if his mother was all right.

On the day of their reading with me, his mother arrived before they did. When I greeted Roy and Yvette at the door, I asked who wanted to go first. "We'd like to go together," said Roy in his broad Scottish accent.

I suggested that the person who had a mother on the other side should go first. I had not yet understood her name — the spirit said it started with a "L" and then she spelled out "M-A-R." That stood for Marshall, which was apparently what Roy's father called her. She said that she had recently passed away from colon cancer. I could tell that this spirit might be feisty on the outside but that she really had a heart of gold.

Roy's mother also told me about her sister, whose name sounded like "Ellen" but started with "H". Roy explained that while everyone called his aunt Ellen, her real name was Helen. Roy's mother further explained that her sister lived in Spain and she made two trips to visit her when she was sick. Roy confirmed that this was the case.

I could tell that the reading was going really well because of Roy and Yvette's enthusiasm. At one point, Roy's mother showed me that she was holding a birthday card for whoever had a birthday in December. Roy stated that it would have been for him.

One night soon after their failed reading, Roy had a vivid dream in which his mother and his aunt appeared. As I described this dream back to him, I could see how moved Roy was to realize I was speaking to his mother. She had helped me describe everything in great detail.

When I later turned to Yvette, I was able to pick up her uncle, grandmother and grandfather. Roy and Yvette were amazed when I was able to give them the correct names for each of them. When her grandmother mentioned the name Sadie, Yvette cringed — Sadie was her middle name. She had always hated it and the only person to use that name was her grandmother!

Her grandmother went on to congratulate

Roy and Yvette on their new house and even described the new sod in the backyard. Roy and Yvette explained that laying the sod had been the first thing that they had done when they moved in. Throughout the reading, Roy's mother kept butting in with more messages. Roy smiled whenever she did — that was just her nature.

After the reading, Roy and Yvette explained that they had come to me with the expectation of being disappointed again. But within two minutes of walking through my door, they knew that this was for real. It especially hit home when I said that Roy's mother had died of cancer. They were overjoyed with the reading and the messages they were given.

Their experience affected them deeply. After their first encounter with a medium, they had continued to hope that they would get the answers they were looking for. They often watched *Crossing Over With John Edwards* on television and planned to go to a taping of the show. But they now had what they needed to confirm their beliefs about the world beyond ours. For his part, Roy says that while he doesn't believe in God, he does believe in an afterlife, a state in which we each become pure energy.

In a later email to me, Roy expressed how he felt that his mother was around him on several occasions before coming to see me. What I said verified that she was there. Though he used to feel strange talking to her, he now feels confident that his mother is listening — he especially feels close to her when he is alone driving in the car.

All this was hard for Roy to take in. While he was here with me, he was careful to write everything down — whenever he reads over his notes now, he still can't believe everything that was said. I am proud to be a part of readings like this. When a reading really helps people, I feel overwhelmed by their enthusiasm and truly privileged to have played a part in their journey towards a higher understanding of life and death.

# 7

# Searching For Meaning

Jamie has a wonderful personality — she is the sort of person who is always quick to laugh. But when she first came to see me, she was struggling to come to terms with the death of her mother the year before. She was searching for a way to connect with her.

Jamie was a self-confessed "non-believer." Not only did she not believe in God but she also didn't believe in an afterlife. Growing up she didn't go to church because of her mother's beliefs. When her mother was a child, she was inseparable from her younger sister. Her death at the age of 11 left Jamie's mother devastated. "If there was a God," she asked, "how could He be so cruel to take my sister away?" From that moment on, she refused not only to attend church but also to believe.

Jamie heard about me through a friend and decided that she didn't have anything to lose. She was in a state of turmoil. She wanted to believe in an afterlife for her mother's sake but she did not know whether or not she could come to terms with the idea of a heaven.

As I started the reading, I noticed a lady in the background. I could tell that she was close to Jamie but I thought she was probably a sister or an aunt rather than her mother. I listened to a few other spirits before getting back to her. When I listened to that spirit the second time, I could tell that she actually was Jamie's mother. She told me to say, "It had been me with the light bulb."

Jamie was floored at what I had just said. Apparently she had forgotten the incident herself until I had mentioned it. Jamie had been home alone crying a few months before. She did not know if her mother was okay and felt lost and in pain. As she stormed up the stairs, she said out loud to herself, "If there is a God, I want a sign." Just then she threw out her hand to flick on the hall light. There was a sudden bang and flash as the light bulb popped. She noticed what had happened but was unsure whether this was the sign that she had asked for.

I explained to Jamie how souls try to communicate with us. "Since a soul leaves the constraints of a body," I said, "they sometimes use items around us to communicate. Your mother is pure energy and she would have found it easy to use electricity — and, in particular, that light bulb — to send you a sign."

Her mother was not finished yet. She wanted

Jamie to burn her candles. I thought it was probably some religious symbol but Jamie laughed. "My
mother made beeswax candles," she explained. Even
when her mother was alive, she would tell Jamie to
burn her candles. As soon as she had used up those
ones, her mother would make her more. Jamie
insisted on saving them because they were too pret-
ty. Especially now, Jamie felt they were too precious
to burn.

Before her mother left, she showed me that
she was holding a baby. Jamie immediately recognized this baby as her brother's baby, who died
when he was six days old. She assured Jamie that
she was taking good care of her nephew.

Another spirit was her grandfather. I got the
name Seth and saw a flag with a blue background
with yellow lines. Jamie confirmed that Seth was
her grandfather's name and that he was from
Sweden. He told us that whenever she drove her
car, he always traveled in the backseat. He likes to
watch over her while she is driving to make sure
she is safe. "That's just like him," Jamie said.

Many more visitors arrived, including her
other grandfather and her great-grandmothers. She
received messages that she would marry in the near
future. Jamie was surprised to hear this since she
had no intention of getting married any time soon.

## Jamie's Visitors

Four years passed before Jamie returned for another reading. Since I see so many people, I didn't realize that we had met before. But when I told her that her mother was already waiting for her, Jamie laughed. She explained that it was typical of her to note that she was late, even if it was only by five minutes.

Her mother communicated that she had cancer in the stomach region. Jamie further clarified that her mother had colon cancer. Her mother also told her that she visited her often and even said that she really likes the dress that Jamie has chosen to get married in.

Soon I picked up another gentleman beside her mother. After I said "Michael," I changed my mind and said, "Mike." He kept pointing to his head so I thought he may have died due to a head trauma. Jamie remembered that it must have been her fiancé's father. His name was Michael but all his life he went by Mike. He had died in a water-skiing accident. He had fallen in shallow water and hit his head on the bottom. He went on to say that he had five children from his first marriage but that he regularly visits all his children.

I kept telling Jamie how popular she was because more and more souls kept showing up. There was everyone from her father's sister Gayle to her girlfriend's mother, in addition to some repeat visitors, such as her great-grandmothers and nephew.

Shortly before she left, Jamie reminded me that she had been to see me before. She explained how she had not believed in God before she came and how she now believes in Him and in the after-life. When she first came, she said that she was shocked, then scared of the idea of souls around her. First she felt happy that they were well, then sad that they were not alive any more. When she left, she felt at peace and was glad to know. The experience reassured her.

**8**

# A Lost Love

"I have a father with me — did your father pass away?"

The young woman in front of me shook her head.

"Did your father-in-law pass away?"

She shook her head again. Something was not quite right with the information I was being given. I decided to leave it with her to see if I could get the right information.

The figure stepped back for a moment. In his place, an aunt and a grandmother stepped forward. The grandmother told me about her four grandchildren so that Susan would know who was speaking. Then they gave me a message that they were specifically watching and giving support to her aunt's son Vincent and his new wife. Susan did not fully understand this message until two weeks later at a family function, when she discovered that her cousin and his wife were expecting a child.

The father figure stepped forward again. "Who is the 'R'?" I asked Susan. "Robert? Robbie? Rob?"

Susan was caught off guard by my statement but the figure kept giving me new information. I needed to let the information flow through me before I forgot.

"Wow," I said, feeling the extent of the relationship, "you guys were close."

"That's my husband," said Susan.

It was my turn to be taken aback. Susan looked too young to have lost a husband. My heart went out to her. Apparently, her husband had gone by all the names that I had listed. She had hoped he would be here but was afraid to hope too much.

As I continued to give her the messages from Rob, I could tell that it meant so much to her to know that he was still around, nearly 20 months after his death.

"You have two children," I said. I realized this was why the figure registered as a father. Rob then started to tell me about his "blond-haired babies," his special name for his children. He told me about his youngest child, a daughter, and how she talks openly about all her memories of him. He kept repeating that she was always talking. Susan laughed when I said, "She really talks a lot."

Susan said his daughter was at peace with what has happened to him. But his son was bottling up the pain and not talking about it. My heart went out to Susan.

Between what Rob said and what Susan shared with me, I discovered what happened the night that he passed away. A sudden asthma attack caused Rob to gasp for air. Susan went to call 911 and while she was on the phone giving them all the information that they needed, Rob collapsed. He had tried to go outside to get some air and passed out from the lack of oxygen. When he fell, he hit his head on the dryer so Susan had found him lying face down.

Rob explained how Susan had screamed on the phone when she heard him fall. It woke up the children and their son and daughter rushed out of bed to find out what was happening.

His daughter, who was only 6 at the time, stayed on the phone while Susan did CPR on her husband — the ambulance arrived half an hour later. Her eight-year-old son was in the terrible position of having to relay information between Susan and his sister. Rob told me how his son was playing the images of that night over and over again like a movie in his mind. He suggested to Susan that she try to help him remember all of the happier memories. Rob suggested that Susan try to talk to him while they were driving because if Susan was not looking at her son, he would find it easier to open up. A couple days later, Susan did exactly that and he began to talk more openly about his feelings.

Susan felt very moved that Rob chose to originally identify himself to me as a father. In life, he had been a very involved father and left some precious memories with his children. Since they were very young, he sang special songs to each of his children — "Brown Eyed Girl" to his daughter and "Stuck In The Middle With You" to his son. He asked Susan to make sure that his children remember all the little things that he did for them, like those songs.

## He Never Left

Rob turned his attention to Susan. He showed me how evenings were the hardest for her. During the day, she could put on a brave face. But at night when the kids were in bed, she found it very difficult to cope. I knew Susan felt comforted when I told her Rob watches over her at night and even tucks her in when she falls asleep on the couch.

"He wishes you a Happy Birthday," I said. The week before she came to see me, Susan had just celebrated her thirtieth birthday. She was glad to know Rob had watched her when she went out for dinner with friends.

"He has a strong presence," I told Susan. "Everyone knew when he walked in a room. He was so jovial and eager to make people laugh.

"I do not know if this is going to make sense but he is telling me that you made him chase you."

A smile crossed Susan's face and I knew that it made sense. I then went on to describe their first date. They had met in high school and married four years later. Susan had been the first girl that made Rob "chase" her. He explained how he had kept calling and calling her to get her to go out with him. Susan later said how this story had been a very defining moment for her because not many people knew how they met. "Chase" was very much Rob's choice of word.

Rob then showed me a tree that he was looking after. He was watching over all the trees that they planted in their yard a year ago, but there was one to which he was paying particular attention. He even showed me how he watched Susan whenever she looked at it from their kitchen window. Susan explained how she had got a gift certificate for a tree shortly after Rob passed away. She didn't tell anyone that she had gone out, gotten the tree and planted it so that she could see it from the kitchen sink.

Shortly after Rob had passed away, they moved into the new house that they had just built. Rob wanted to paint it all white but Susan loved colours too much to allow that to happen. Susan told me how she had chosen colours for every room and the only thing that ended up being white was their daughter's ceiling. Rob had a special message for his wife about colours on the other side. He tried to explain but words failed him. Finally, he could only say that Susan wouldn't know what blue, green and orange really were until she had seen them there.

## A Special Message

"You had a dream not long ago which was very comforting to you," I said. "It really helped you."

Susan's eyes welled up with tears as she told me how she had just woken up when Jamie appeared. She could see the outline of his face, his eyes and his eyebrows. He didn't say anything at all — he just looked at her. At first she thought she was still sleeping but she looked at him from every direction for what seemed like hours. Then suddenly he was gone.

I told her that he would visit her again in her sleep. Susan later told me that that evening when she went to bed, she was so exhausted and so drained that she slept like a log. Ever since his death she had suffered from insomnia and could only sleep for two or three hours at a time. However, the night after our reading, she fell into a deep sleep for six hours. During that time, Rob came to visit. He was a very romantic man and always hugged her as soon as he arrived home. That night, Susan felt Rob give her an incredible hug. She cherished that feeling — it reminded her of the embraces he gave her when he was alive.

"He wants you to quit dwelling on his death. You need to move on." I waited for Rob's statement to sink in before I continued. "You have not buried him. He says if you want to bury him then go ahead. If you want to continue to carry him around, then he says you can do that too. It does not matter to him."

Within the last few months, Diana had been unsure over what to do. When Jamie died, she placed his ashes in a specially made urn. She had not told anyone but she had thought about burying the urn on the first day of spring. But she was scared to do that because then she would have another day to mourn him. She had already decided to wait until his death in September before doing anything with the urn.

For the last two years, the urn had taken Rob's place on the family's annual male bonding weekend, in which all the men would go out to camp and hunt. Since Rob's death, they continued to come by her house and borrow the urn, which they strapped to the backseat. One year while they were hunting, her uncle asked for a sign to prove that Rob was with them. When they turned a corner in the road, a deer was standing in the middle of the road. When her uncle tells this story, he always says that he should have asked for a larger deer.

**Reconnecting**

Rob went on to say that he had so many people with him, he was not lonely. He kept mentioning a younger person with a name that started with "M". Susan didn't know who that could be so I left it with him. Rob then brought up the name Jimmy or Jim. Susan still could not place those names either.

"Rob said to bring up your sister-in-law and that she would know."

Susan was stunned. She had been careful not to say that she had brought her sister-in-law Violet to the reading and that she was waiting downstairs.

Violet seemed very apprehensive when she came upstairs.

"We were just talking with your brother Rob," I told her. I could tell that Violet wanted to connect with her brother but she couldn't believe what was happening.

The first message Rob gave her was how proud he was for her going back to school at 28. He then brought up the names again. Violet almost immediately knew about the "M" — it was for Morgan, a nephew from her husband's side of the family who passed away when he was seven. Rob and Morgan had only met on the other side. Jim, meanwhile, was a neighbour who lived down the road from them when they were kids. He had died around the time of his graduation. Rob wanted Violet to know that everyone was all right.

He then showed me a room with teddy bears lined up all around it. "Is that your daughter's room?" I asked Violet. She shook her head so I asked for more information. "The room was pink." Still no recollection. "Who is Charlotte?"

"That's my daughter's middle name," replied Susan. She hadn't immediately recognized it because he was describing her daughter's room in the trailer where they lived while they were building their new home. It had been a very pink room and she had lined all her teddy bears up against the walls.

Rob had so many more things to tell everyone but I could tell that everyone was exhausted, even Rob. Despite her fatigue, Susan was finding it hard to leave. She had finally found a little piece of Rob again. After such a long time of remembering and not being with him, she finally felt connected to him again.

Since her reading, people have told her that she looks happier. Susan says it is good to know that Rob is with her all the time.

Susan's youth struck a chord with me. Society

does not know how to deal with young widows. People always say that losing a child is the greatest loss and we can generally relate easier to that kind of grief. People forget that she lost a husband and that her children lost a father.

**9**

**Christmas Spirit**

It was December 23 and the Christmas rush was in full gear at my house. I still had plenty to do, like wrapping gifts, shopping for groceries and doing all of the cleaning and tidying before my guests arrived for Christmas dinner.

As I was writing my to-do list, the telephone rang. I was hoping that it was someone calling to help me but I knew that it was not the case. The young woman on the other end asked if she could come for a reading before Christmas. I explained that while I did not have time to fit her in, I would certainly make time if she were to call me in the New Year.

She said that she understood but went on to say that she was not looking forward to the holidays. She said she was really "at the end of her rope." At that moment, I knew I needed to make the time to see her. I told her that if 9:30 that evening was not too late, she could come over. She readily agreed.

She arrived on my doorstep at precisely 9:30 p.m. I asked her to relax on the couch while I made us tea — my usual warm up for a reading. As I was running the water, I had the sense of a man with me there in the kitchen. He gave me a warm, fuzzy feeling, one of great love and comfort. But it wasn't for me — it was for Mariah.

I popped my head around the corner. "I have a man here," I told Mariah, "for you in spirit. He says his name is Harry."

By the look on her face, I could tell that she recognized him.

"That's my father," she said. "His name was actually Airry, a Dutch form of Harry."

"He's right here," I said, "and he wants you to know that he loves and is always with you. He tells me that he died of a heart attack." She said that was true. "He wants to tell you of a young man that is with him. I think he was in an accident, a motor vehicle accident."

At this, Mariah's eyes began to fill with tears. This was why she was here.

"He says his name was David," I said.

Mariah looked at me with an expression of disbelief and broke down. Her husband David had died nine months ago in an accident between his truck and a drunk driver in another car. Mariah had two sons — one was 3, the other only 18 months old. She was facing her first Christmas without her husband.

David proceeded to tell Mariah through me that he was fine, with her father and he was watching over her and the boys all the time. He told Mariah that it was all right to move on with her life, to see other people. He wanted her to be happy.

He also told her that he was especially close to Don and Dino, that he visited them often. I asked Julie if she knew who these people were. Mariah was flabbergasted — David's mother was Donna and his brother is Dean. Mariah said she could feel David's presence — the energy in the room was unmistakable.

I then gave Mariah David's final parting message: "Merry Christmas and Happy Anniversary."

"Our wedding anniversary is between Christmas and New Year's Eve," she said in amazement.

We stood at the door and hugged the longest, strongest hug as she thanked me over and over again. She had found some peace. I told her to get home and have a wonderful Christmas with those beautiful sons of hers. I knew she could do it.

As I closed the door and watched her leave, I thanked God for this beautiful soul I had the opportunity to meet and help. This was the best Christmas gift ever. Such was the warmth running through me, I felt like I would never need to do another reading. I felt truly blessed.

# 10

# Discovering A Mother's Love

"I feel that your mother has passed over," I said to Olivia, who seemed to me to be a sweet young woman in her early twenties.

"Not really," she replied in a polite, soft voice.

I was a bit confused by her response. Maybe it would make more sense if I gave her more information. "She is giving me the name Ivy."

"Yes, that is my mother," Olivia replied.

Her statement really confused me. I was sure that the spirit in front of me was Olivia's mother Ivy. After pausing for a moment to be sure I was getting the right information, I repeated what I knew. "I've got your mother right here. She says that she passed away a long time ago in a car accident. I don't even know if you remember her."

"I do and I don't."

"She is showing me a baby," I said. "I think it is you. You were young when the accident happened."

"Yes," said Olivia, "I was nine months old."

"When the accident happened you were in the car with her. It was late afternoon when it happened. You and your mother had just finished getting the groceries. Your mother was badly injured but you were all right because you were in your car seat."

Though Olivia could not remember any of these details, she confirmed them later with her father.

"I am picking up that you visit your mother."

This too seemed strange. I felt that she wasn't visiting a gravesite but rather visiting Ivy in person. I couldn't get my head around the information I was being given.

Finally, it dawned on me. "Your mother is in the hospital — she is hooked up to machines in a coma."

"Yes," said Olivia as tears started to pour down her cheeks. "She has been in a coma for 23 years."

I had never expected that, but everything made sense. I realized the gravity of what was taking place. I always thought that I could communicate with people in a coma but until that moment I never knew for sure. It made sense to me that the soul would slip in and out even if her body had not died. I imagine it would be very much like the out-of-body experiences I had when I was younger. People who have spent time around coma patients say that they seem present sometimes, then not at other times. If their souls are slipping in and out of their physical bodies, this would explain that feeling.

It dawned on me that Olivia's mother Ivy had been in a coma for 23 years — that's a very long time to be in a coma. If Olivia had been nine months old when the accident happened, she would be 24 or 25 right now.

Growing up, Olivia heard only a few details about the accident and about her mother. Otherwise, it was as if she never existed. She had never known her mother as a conscious person, which meant she did not know what her mother's personality was like. Olivia would visit her in the hospital periodically, but less and less so as the years went by. It was so hard on Olivia to see someone that looked so much like her but whom she couldn't communicate with or learn about.

"Ivy's actual spirit left her on impact," I told Olivia. "What you saw was just a body. She may have been lying there but she has been around you all the time."

Olivia seemed comforted by this realization. She also felt closer to her to know that she had been around her. This experience was very emotional for her because it was the first chance she had to talk to her mother. "She is so proud of you," I told her. "She was there at your high school and college graduation for spiritual support."

Her mother obviously had so much love for her. And as Olivia was able to connect with her, I could also see the love she had for Ivy begin to grow.

Olivia had been an only child. Even though her father was still alive, she went to live with her grandparents after Ivy's accident. It was really the best option because of how hard it was for her father to be a single parent while trying to work on his farm. She still saw him everyday. When her father remarried when Olivia was 5, Olivia moved back in with him and eventually had two younger sisters.

"Ivy is glad that he remarried," I said. "He could not have picked a better mother to help raise you. But your father has to let go of his guilt — he did not do anything wrong. Your grandparents are also still alive. I feel that they are the ones having a hard time letting go."

At the time of the accident, they refused to believe that Ivy would not recover. They refused to give up hope even though nothing could be done. Because of her grandparents' insistence to keep Ivy alive, Olivia's father had to divorce her mother before being able to remarry. After the divorce, her grandparents became Ivy's legal guardian. When Olivia turned 18, her mother became her responsibility.

"You don't know what to do, do you?"

Maureen slowly shook her head as tears continued to roll down her face. I could tell that this decision had been a heavy burden. Shortly after turning 18, Olivia told her grandparents that it was not fair to put her in this position and she signed the legal rights back to them.

"Your mother says that she came through to let you know that you can let her go completely," I reassured her. "She says she is not ever going to come back and be conscious again. She is ready to die so whenever you're ready, she is too."

Olivia had never felt any attachment to her mother before her reading. "I have never known her," she told me, "but she must have had a lot of love for me to come through or even want to come through." By talking to her, she was able to get a sense of what she was like. It was the first time that Ivy felt like she knew her mother.

Olivia came back to see me a few times over the following year. Near the end of my time with Olivia, her mother contracted pneumonia. If not treated, the pneumonia would cause other infections and eventually lead to death. At that point her grandparents, knowing how Olivia felt, decided to let nature take its course. Ivy passed away in September of 2001.

# 11

## An Uncertain Past

"I'm seeing a car accident," I told Elise. "He is saying it was not his fault."

But there was something confusing about this reading that I could not put my finger on. I had talked to many people whose loved ones had died in car accidents. Such readings are usually straightforward.

My reading for Elise had started out like a typical reading. When she first arrived, I could see in her face that she had been carrying around a great pain for a long time. In fact, she had been suffering this weight since she was four years old.

After giving her a glass of water and inviting her to sit down, I immediately picked up her father, William. Beside him was his brother. I saw him in a uniform and he told me that he had died in the war. Elise had never met him but she had heard about him and verified that what I said was true.

Another figure with her father was a baby boy. He did not really identify himself but I picked up that he had passed away a long time ago in a tragedy. Her father then talked about Elise's siblings, one sister and two brothers, before telling me about the car accident.

Once I mentioned the accident, Elise immediately asked, "How did he die?"

"He is telling me about a car accident," I said, "but he is saying that it was not his fault. It happened in the 1950s. There was a turn in the road and then the car went over the embankment and hit what appears to be a tree. He was found in the driver's seat and was severely injured. I see three other people in the car. They were barely injured from the accident and walked away with only a few bumps and bruises."

His injuries seemed too extreme — I could tell that the impact was not enough to have hurt him so badly, let alone kill him.

Tears had been pouring down Elise's face ever since I started to talk about the accident. Something still seemed to not quite fit. At the time of the tragedy, she was only 4 so all her information about the accident was secondhand. I realized that she was trying to dig into the past to figure out what had happened.

"Something is missing here," I said. "You have many questions. I see you doing research. I see you looking in two newspapers, a large one and a small one."

"Yes," said Elise, "I found articles about the

accident in two newspapers. One was a local news-paper and the other was a larger newspaper."

"I also see that you talked to an official."

Elise explained that she tracked down the policeman who had originally investigated the accident, but her enquiries had yielded no new information. She also had another question for me: "What are the statutes of limitations on murder?"

I did not know what to say to her. Whatever had happened had made a deep impact on her. The mystery surrounding her father's death had hung over her since she was a young child and I felt sorry that she had to go through any of this. I explained that I was not a lawyer but that I did not think there was a statute of limitation on murder.

Just at that moment, I picked up Elise's moth-er, Dorothy. "I feel that she passed away almost at the same time," I told Elise, "but I do not see her in the car. I see your mother in the kitchen doubled over. She was carrying a baby. I also see her in the hospital. I feel that she died of a miscarriage or abdominal surgery. The condition appeared to be something of a female nature because it was in her abdomen. She is showing me dirty medical instru-ments."

I could tell that Dorothy had been in severe pain. "Had she just had a baby?"

Elise shook her head. I realized that Dorothy

had died of a botched abortion. Dorothy told me that she and William were so poor, they were barely managing to feed the four children — all of whom were under 6 — they already had. She couldn't bear the thought of having another baby, especially one so soon after her last.

Dorothy knew a woman in another town who had done many abortions in the kitchen of her home. However neither woman knew that Dorothy was carrying twins. The woman only managed to do a partial abortion — the other fetus was missed.

Elise's mother had gone to this woman's house in the morning and had the abortion before returning home to her kids again that afternoon. When Dorothy was making dinner that evening, she doubled over and died almost instantly. Her mother kept showing me the dirty instruments — something no one else had known about     because the hemorrhage that killed her was partially caused by an infection.

I could see that the babies had been boys — I saw one with Elise's father earlier in the reading and the other with Dorothy when she first appeared.

Though I wanted to focus more on her mother, Elise was already fairly clear on the details of her awful death. It was still a relief to hear exactly what had happened. When her mother passed away, she left a very young family behind, one that was ill-equipped to handle the car accident seven months later.

I asked Elise's father William for more information about his death. He told me again that the accident wasn't his fault. I could see again that there were other people — two women — at the site. Her father also appeared to me in very rumpled clothes.

"Did your father just come from work? His clothes are rumpled."

Elise shook her head. William then showed me he had been drinking that night. I could tell that he was a regular drinker, but he had sunk deeper into alcoholism after losing his wife. When William showed me his fists, I suddenly realized what had happened. "He was in a fight!" I exclaimed.

The full details began to emerge. I could see a small, typical Western Canadian town, the sort of place where everyone knew everyone else. William had been a slightly hostile person to begin with, but his grief over his wife left him depressed and over-wrought. There had been a fight that rolled out of a small hotel and into the parking lot. I saw a gash across William's head that started at the top and travelled across his forehead to his right eye and onto his right cheek.

"It looked like he was hit with a tire iron," I

told Elise. "I see the man who did it — he did not mean to kill him. The fight just got out of control. He grabbed a tire iron and struck your father.

"I also see two women. They had been drinking in the bar with the men. They helped the man load your father into the car. I cannot see who was driving but they put him into the driver's seat. There was no way he could have driven the car even before being struck — he had been drinking too much."

I then saw them drive the car off the embankment, making it seem as if a car accident had taken place.

But there was another important revelation: one of the ladies was still alive. Unfortunately, we couldn't figure out who she was because the description I gave did not mean anything to Elise.

Elise explained that there had always been doubts about how her father died. What I said confirmed her suspicions that he had been killed before the accident. At the end of the reading, I saw that Elise's pain had been lifted. She went away with a new peace of mind.

# 12

# A Travelling Companion

As I was driving home from Drumheller late one night, I felt a presence in the car with me. I felt tired and drained from doing readings all day so the last thing I wanted was to talk. The only thing on my mind was getting home safely to my children and having a nice warm bath before bed.

The presence came around me shortly after I started to make my way home. It felt like a young, male energy, one I did not recognize as a family member or friend. Fortunately he did not seem to want to talk or have any message for me at that time. I figured that the significance of it would be made apparent in time. I drove on in silence.

I had taken a shortcut on a back road so the only sound that could be heard for miles was my car. All I could see were my headlights on the roughly paved road ahead of me. If I looked to the side, I could just make out the barbwire fence running parallel to the road.

When I came to a T-intersection, I paused before turning. I felt that over to the left that there must be a memorial. I couldn't actually see it because of the darkness but it just felt like it was there. My passenger remained silent and I continued my drive home. As I entered the Calgary city limits, he quietly left my car.

Eight days later, I was doing a message service at the Spiritualist church. I was particularly drawn toward a family of three. I narrowed in on the father and gave him a message about his work from his grandmother.

After the service, his wife asked me for a business card and booked a reading. When they arrived two days later, I immediately picked up on a spirit named Zachary. Zachary told me that he was their son and that he had passed away suddenly and traumatically, perhaps in a vehicle accident. He then began to describe the details.

Zachary had been out drinking with his friends. He got into his truck and started toward home. It was late at night on a gravel road. He was surprised by the sight of a truck coming in the opposite direction. He was going too fast and swerved off the road.

I felt that Zachary had died instantly. Because it was such a rural road and the accident took place late at night, his body was not found until much later. When he showed me the location of where it happened, I realized he had been the one in the car with me. Zachary told me that his friends had placed a makeshift memorial at that intersection, the same place where I had paused.

Zachary was his parents' only son and his death weighed heavily on their hearts. Nothing had been moved from his room. He showed me drawers that were still filled with his stuff. He told them that they could go through his room. He also showed me the sheets on the bed. His mother had washed his sheets but otherwise placed them exactly as they had been when Zachary was alive. His mother would go and sit there. "Whenever you are ready," he told his parents through me, "it's okay to go through my stuff."

He also gave them the names of his grandfather and grandmother and it was a relief for his parents to learn that Zachary was not alone on the other side.

The reading was extremely powerful for me because of the overwhelming grief I felt from his family, who had lost him only a few months before. When given the knowledge that he was still a part of their lives (and always would be), they began to heal.

**13**

## A New Take On Life

*I would like to say that I remember the story of every person who visits me. Unfortunately, my memory is not perfect. While writing this book, I tried to recall stories that helped me develop as a medium or ones that others might be able to relate to. It was not until Kathryn called me as I was writing this section that I remembered her amazing story. Only she can relate all the details and complexities that you need in order to fully understand what she and her family have endured over the last few years. Here is Kathryn's story in her own voice.*

We had lost our son David in very traumatic circumstances. He died shortly before the beginning of a court case in which his wife Carmen was tried for embezzled funds from their company. During his three years of marriage, not only did she destroy the business that he created but she betrayed his trust by cheating on him and lying to all of us.

Carmen had come from a turbulent family where divorce was commonplace. We tried to make her feel like she was a part of our close-knit family. We did everything we could to make her feel welcome and loved. After she married David, we trusted her with everything. Little did we know that she only married our son for monetary gain. At the end of their marriage, she succeeded in causing the financial ruin of not only David but also the whole family. She had used our love against us.

On the day the court case was to begin — February 11 — we discovered that David had taken his life. Unfortunately, none of us had time to properly mourn his death because of the legal proceedings and lifestyle changes resulting from our financial ruin. It would take us many years to deal with his death.

As if losing our son was not enough, both my husband and I had to find employment and start the process of rebuilding our lives. Carmen made things very difficult for us. She sold possessions that we had stored at our son's house and denied us access to items that had no monetary value, such as childhood pictures of David.

Over the next five years, we did everything that everyone suggests to cope with the death of a loved one. We attended grief courses and spoke to counsellors but found that none of this was enough. Then someone mentioned mediums, and Kim in particular. When our daughter Rachael went to see her, she was blown away. The revelations and the details of everything left Rachael with no doubts that Kim was speaking directly to David.

Over the following months I watched how our daughter's visit with Kim helped her heal. Rachael even began to feel positive about the future. Still, it took me many months before I had the courage to see Kim. I thought I knew what to expect, but nothing Rachel could say would prepare me for such a powerful experience. Kim was able to describe everything about David — from his hair and eye colour to the clothes that he was wearing when he took his life. She even described his funeral and facts that were only revealed during the court case.

Without me needing to say anything, Kim explained how David had accomplished everything he had sought out to do and how his business had been his dream. She then went on to describe how David's wife Carmen had taken his love, his new home, his construction business and even his dog. She even explained how his wife had made sure to finish embezzling the money we had invested in David's business just a few months before we were due to be paid out.

Kim then acknowledged all the personal items that Carmen had denied us, such as David's school pictures. I was truly amazed when she asked about the classroom handprint, which was one of the few items Carmen returned to us, though when we received it, it had been broken into pieces.

When I left that first visit with Kim, I felt exhausted. Yet the comfort she provided was undeniable. It was such a huge relief to know that David was all right. We never questioned why he took his life — we knew what he was going through — so this experience was more about connecting with him and easing our pain at losing him.

I shared everything that Kim had said with my family and friends. It was amazing to all of us — surely it was impossible for anyone to know all these things.

My husband Bob eventually built up the courage to see Kim. David's death was particularly hard on him because they had worked so closely together. During his reading, many of the same things happened as they did with me. Kim told Bob things that no one could have known, such as the fact that his best friend died of cancer a month after David passed away.

As we continued to visit Kim, she gave us more and more amazing news. Four years before my daughter Rachael had children, Kim predicted that she would have a boy first, then a girl two years later. Kim went into great detail with each child. She predicted that David would be part of the first child's name, as indeed he was. The boy would be named Andrew David (I'll tell you more about him later). Kim also said the girl's name would be Amy Lynn, which was the name that Rachael had already chosen. Kim then predicted the exact day that Amy Lynn was born and said she would weigh just under six pounds — when Amy was born, she weighed five pounds and 12 ounces.

Kim has given us so much comfort. Time and time again she has given us proof that we're not crazy. We believe and trust in her completely.

**Proof That David Lives On**

Some people might be tempted to plan their lives according to Kim's predictions. But much of what she predicted for us was forgotten about until it occurred. That's what happened when we visited Kim and David told us that we would leave home on a holiday, our first in years. He said that we needed a vacation and predicted that we would go somewhere warm.

Neither of these statements seemed like much of a prediction but it was what he said next that really stood out. He predicted that on the first evening after we arrived, we would be sitting outside and hear a train whistle. He said that whistle would be him.

A few years later, my husband and I went to

the condo we had just purchased. We had never been there before and on our way there, we crossed a railroad track but didn't think twice about it. On our first night there, we went out onto the patio while the sun was setting at 9 o'clock. Within minutes of sitting down, a train whistle from the railroad tracks nearby blasted through the silence. At that instant, I remembered what Kim had said and knew that it was David. It was such an incredible moment.

Prior to my daughter's wedding, Kim told us that Rachael would arrive at her wedding in a huge white car. I was a little annoyed at this because it didn't sound much like a prediction — after all, most people use a white limousine on their wedding day. But shortly before the happy day, my husband and I purchased a brand-new white station wagon. When my husband and I picked up Rachael on her wedding day, we all remembered Kim's prediction.

Another event that she described was about a visit to David's gravesite at Christmas time. Prior to this, we had been denied access to it by his former wife. Rachael bought a three-foot-high Christmas tree and planned to place it beside Jeff's gravesite because Christmas was his favourite time of year. Through Kim, David had told us that he loved it but he wanted us to make new traditions without him. We decided to take Rachael's tree with us to the condo. When we talked to Kim later, she described the sight of the tree in our condo, proving that he had shared Christmas with us.

One of the most remarkable revelations was about Rachael's son, Andrew David. When Kim described what he would be like, she could have been describing David. If we put baby pictures of David beside pictures of Andrew, the only way we can tell them apart is from the clothes they wear. Their personalities are also very similar. David had been outgoing and funny. In school, he was an above-average student and had been a great athlete — he also showed some musical talent. Even at Andrew's young age, we can tell that he has these same attributes.

At times we've seen Andrew stare out into space and then burst out laughing. When he was an infant, we would often find him babbling and laughing in his crib. Kim told us that these are the times when David is communicating to Andrew. There is some evidence that this is true — Andrew was probably the only two-year-old who knew the difference between a Bobcat, a Backhoe and a Trackhoe before he ever said the word "car." It is just not normal for such a young child to know so much about construction vehicles unless someone like David had taken the time to teach him.

There are just so many stories that there can never be enough time to tell them. All I can say is that what we've gone through with Kim is amazing. Whenever any of our friends or family members have been to see her, David has been there, too, even when Kim had no prior knowledge that the person had any connection to us.

She's made believers out of even our family's sceptics and all of us have found her healing power unquestionable. It's a great gift to know that we can go to her whenever we feel the need. It has been such a comfort to know that David is around us and that we are able to communicate with him. We know without a doubt that our loved one is there.

# 14

# Becoming Clairvoyant Kim

I thought about going on the radio years before I performed my first reading. The idea came to me when I was pregnant with my first daughter. I had the radio on while I was doing some house-work one afternoon. I was listening to a phone-in show when a psychic came on. This was a novel idea at the time — this was before the days of infomercial for psychic hotlines. Spiritualism was neither well-known nor highly regarded.

When I heard the psychic, I noted the unique-ness of the concept. I even called the show. I could not believe it when my call went through. I told the psychic that I was expecting a baby soon. I wanted to know if the baby was healthy and also what sex it was. He replied that the baby would be a healthy baby boy. A few months later, I became the proud mother of a healthy baby girl. The radio idea stuck anyway.

As my work as a medium grew, I often thought about going on the radio. I know better than most people that reoccurring thoughts should be interpreted as special messages. Finally, I decided to do something about it. One day I just opened the phone book to the letter "C" for Canada and Calgary and the name of 66 CFR popped out at me. I dialled the radio station's general number. It turned out to be the number for a group of three different stations. I explained to the receptionist what I did and what I wanted. "You need to speak with Tara Connors," she said. She put me through to Tara's voicemail and I left a message.

Weeks passed and I didn't hear back so I did not think any more about it. Then, over a month later, the phone rang just after I started a bath for my daughter. The call display revealed that it was 66 CFR and I instantly became flustered. I did not know if I wanted to answer it.

Tara Connors and Pat O'Bryan were on the line and eager to talk to me about my idea. I was taken aback by Tara's enthusiasm, so much so that I was unsure whether I could actually do it. But both she and Pat were so encouraging, I could not refuse. During our call, Tara was so excited, she completely forgot to ask me for my last name or to ask if I had any credentials.

Ten days later, I showed up at 7 a.m. to appear on 66 CFR's morning show. Since I wasn't sure how well I would do, I hadn't told anyone that I would be on except for my mother and a single friend — I was scared I would embarrass myself. Pat was there in the booth and instantly made me feel at ease. He explained that in the run-up to the show he had not known what to call me since the station did not have my last name. He hoped I did not mind being called Clairvoyant Kim. I said, "Sure, that sounds great." I would try out a few other names, like "Calgary's radio psychic," but when Pat became ill and died, I decided that I would always use Clairvoyant Kim.

Everything happened so quickly. After Pat announced on the radio who I was and what I did, the phones began to ring off the hook. During a break after the second reading, Tara asked me if I wanted to make this a regular event. After that, I started showing up once a month. We even moved my appearance to 6 a.m. due to the volume of calls.

After a year at the station, I began to meet other radio personalities. One morning, I was sitting on the couch in the reception area and Samantha Stevens sat beside me. We started chatting and she asked if I would like to come on her show as well. I began appearing on her midday show on Rock 97 once a month, achieving the same response as I did in the morning.

Christina Rowsell and I met a few months later when I was in the control room with Samantha. When she was on Power 107, she had the city's top-rated morning show for three years — I used to hear it all the time because my daughter would listen to it at top volume. She left to host her own show in Victoria but having missed Calgary she had just returned and was waiting for the right opening.

When she got a new show on Country 105, she asked if I would go on the air with her. Since Country 105 broadcasts not only in Calgary but around the world on the Internet, I had a lot of calls for readings. My radio career has really taken off.

I absolutely love doing all the radio shows and I always get a kick out of people's reactions. Many of the announcers have also become friends so we have great chemistry on the air.

# 15

# Behind the Scenes with Christina

*How did you first meet Kim?*

I was filling in at 66 CFR and my friend Samantha Stevens often told me about the medium who had been coming on her show for the last few months. She said I should pop in one day and meet her. When I walked into the control room, Kim immediately said that I have two grandmothers here in the room. Both of my grandmothers had passed away. She also said that one was taller than the other one. That too was true — one was five-foot-eight and the other was five-foot-two.

Then I asked Kim what their names were, knowing they were both the same. Kim knew that too! Before I had the chance to take everything in, Kim wrote the letter "R" on the table and told me that that was the first letter of the name they shared. My grandmothers were both named Rita.

When I got my show on Country 105, I asked Kim to come on. Now she comes in once a month to do a show. She has been a huge success. People constantly phone the station to ask when she will be on.

*What does Kim do when she performs readings?*
On the show, I instruct the callers to ask one specific question. For instance, someone may ask a question like, "Where is my love life going?" Kim then will look off into the distance. Sometimes, she'll move her head around and blink. I've noticed that her nose will twitch as if she were about to sneeze. Once she starts to reply, she doesn't stop talking. All this information just flows out of her.

Kim's whole process is very interesting on the radio because there is no way to know who is going to call. I'm amazed that she can be so specific and accurate just from a telephone call. Callers cannot believe it. I remember one time when a male caller asked Kim, "Am I going to see my children grow up?" I started to go through all the reasons why someone would ask that — was he going through a divorce or moving away or very ill?

Kim asked him if he had polyps. I could hear how stunned he was. "You're bang on," he said. Kim went on to explain that he was going to be all right and that he would indeed see his children grow up.

*Who are Kim's callers?*
There seems to be two types. Most are amazed by what she says and want her number afterward. Other callers don't like her answers. Those people want Kim to say exactly what they

want to hear. But Kim only says what she knows to be true.

One woman caller said that her boyfriend was married. Before she had time to continue Kim said, "You do not have to be psychic to know that he is not going to leave his wife. Besides, you already know that."

*What do you like about having Kim on your show?*

Kim has an amazing quality that is difficult to describe. Not only does she help people by making them feel at peace with the death of a loved one, but callers trust her. That is a difficult quality to have on the radio yet people seem to be able to tell that she is genuine. So when she tells people that they do not need to worry about those they have lost but should worry about themselves instead, people know that to be true. She makes you feel better that the people we've lost have gone on to a better place.

And becoming such close friends with her has been incredible for me. She is so generous with her gifts. We will be out on a hike or be in her kitchen and out of the blue, she'll say that so-and-so is here. One evening while I was sitting in her kitchen, she asked, "Who is Leonard?" I had never told her my grandfather's name and she went on to describe him. She just blows you away with her abilities.

People are always looking for answers and Kim can help people find them. All the announcers at the station are always being asked when she will be on next. The response to her has been amazing.

# 16

# Reflections

I feel that I have the best job on earth. That's because I cannot believe people actually pay me to do something I enjoy. What's more, it all comes so naturally to me.

And everyday I experience the joy in seeing how what I do helps people. At times, I even get to witness the ways my readings can change them. Reactions are often the same but the results vary from person to person. Some people, like Roy and Zachary's parents, need closure and walk away with a confirmation of an afterlife. Their readings prove to them that their original beliefs in the other side were correct. By contrast, other people, like Jamie, go through a stunning transformation in which they must change their entire concept of God and embrace a new understanding of the world around them.

Sometimes people, like Susan and Mariah, need to reconnect to loved ones who have passed over. They needed to know that their loved ones are safe and still with them. By realizing that their loved ones never really left, they feel at peace with what happened this in turn helps those around them. Their readings have the power to help other people who were not even there. What they learnt has a ripple effect by helping their children start to heal.

Connecting to loved ones and gaining insights from them can be a powerful experience. Olivia never really knew her mother but discovering that her mother loves her and watches over her has helped her feel closer to her — her story still touches me today. Elise needed answers to question surrounding her father's death. Finding the truth alleviated nagging doubts that had plagued her for years.

Another great part of my job is having the opportunity to remove the fears people have about the afterlife. Families and friends find relief knowing that their loved ones are still with them and that the other realm is around us all the time. The story in the chapter entitled "A New Take On Life" is a perfect example of this. Many people also attach a stigma to suicide. When someone takes their own life, it was still that soul's choice as to when they wanted to leave. His or her death is no different from anyone else's — the spirit still finds healing in heaven. It is only those of us who are left behind that struggle with the pain of death.

Sometimes when I do a reading the smallest

things turn out to be the biggest things. By being able to tell a woman that her son had a haircut yesterday or that she visited the dentist a few days before, she can understand that spirits are constantly around us. One time, a soul gave me the scent of peanut butter cookies. I asked the lady with me if she had been making them the day before. That question brought on a flood of tears. She had spent the whole day making twelve dozen cookies for one of her daughter's school fundraisers. She realized that her late husband had been there in the kitchen, watching her.

Even a nickname can help a person fully understand what I am saying. When people ask me what a particular soul used to call them, I put the idea out there. When the correct response comes, the impact is very powerful — suddenly it all just seems to click.

This job is more than I ever hoped or dreamed for. Before I accepted my gifts, I would think, "Why me?" Now I think, "Why not me?" When people ask me if my gift is a burden that wears on me, I tell them that it is the best thing that ever happened to me. I cannot imagine doing anything else. At times, I find it hard to grasp what I do. I even surprise myself. A thought will just come to me. When I ask the person at the reading if what I'm repeating is true, I am amazed when they say that it is.

When I explain what I do to some people, they look at me as if I am from another planet. Yet it feels very natural to me. In some ways, I think it still hasn't hit me that I talk to dead people. All I know is that every reading I do also adds something to my life. It has everything to do with karma and listening to my inner voice. Every time I do a reading, I help people. The more I share my gifts with others, the better my own life becomes. Before I started doing readings, I went through some tough times. Ever since I began to help others, my life has become better and better. Everything just seems to work out for me.

It still has not completely sunk in.